THE ESSENTIAL HANDBOOK TO LECTIN

THE PROTEIN CAUSING INFLAMMATION, DIGESTIVE ISSUES, AND WEIGHT GAIN

BY

EVELYN CARMICHAEL

Evelyn Carmichael

INTRODUCTION

Many people eat a gluten-free diet, but they may not be aware that the real culprit that's responsible for their ill health is in fact a protein known as lectin. This little-known intolerance can cause a wide range of nasty symptoms, from Leaky Gut to Autoimmune Disorders. The good news is that you can help to eliminate those symptoms if you make a few changes to the way that you eat.

If you are one of the thousands of individuals on a gluten free diet but still experiencing the same symptoms that led you to try the diet, you may need to also reduce lectins from your diet. If you did not test positive for a gluten sensitivity, but find you feel a bit better on a gluten free diet, lectin intolerance may also be something you want to consider. Lectins may be responsible for your symptoms and in some cases, may be able to reverse your diagnosis once you decrease them from your diet.

Evelyn Carmichael

This book will look at exactly what lectins are, the relationship with gluten, and exactly how to reduce them from your diet. With a little bit of guidance and determination, you too may start to feel better by changing the way you eat.

The Essential Handbook to Lectin

Evelyn Carmichael

TABLE OF CONTENTS

Introduction 3

Table of Contents 7

Legal Notes 9

Chapter 1. Lectin and the Gluten Connection 11

Chapter 2. Why Are Lectins Harmful To Your Body? 17

Chapter 3. Low and High Lectin Foods 27

Chapter 4. How to Reduce Lectin Counts in High Lectin Foods 41

Chapter 5. Reducing Lectin From Your Diet 49

Chapter 6. Making the Switch to Low-Lectin Foods 57

Excerpt of The Essential Handbook to Turmeric and Ginger 65

About The Author 75

Other Books By Evelyn Carmichael 77

References 81

Author Note 83

Evelyn Carmichael

LEGAL NOTES

Evelyn Carmichael

CHAPTER 1. LECTIN AND THE GLUTEN CONNECTION

These days it seems that many individuals are eliminating gluten from their diet. Autoimmune Disease such as Celiac's, Hashimoto's, Rheumatoid Arthritis, and others are on the rise with nearly all individuals trying to reduce inflammation in their body and believe gluten is the culprit. For many, it is, but it may only be one piece in a much larger puzzle.

We know that some people claim to be gluten-intolerant, and state they feel better after eating a gluten-free diet, but there could be another underlying issue that is only partly

11

gluten-related. In fact, the larger and in many cases underlying issue for the diseases themselves is actually something called lectin.

What is lectin?

Lectin is a protein, and it can be found in plants that need to defend themselves. If you're a keen gardener, or you simply know a little bit about plants, you'll know that plants, like any prey, feel the need to defend themselves from birds, insects, and anything that wants to eat them. Plants contain lectin, which the birds, insects etc. eat, which in turn makes him ill. This is nature's way of defending itself, and telling the birds, insects etc. not to eat them again. Think of lectin as a low-level toxin that the plant uses to make its prey not want to touch it again.

The fact of the matter is that when we decide to eat these plants, we are not as immune to the lectin as we might like to think we are. When many of us eat plants that contain lectin, we can start to feel unwell, perhaps we take an indigestion tablet, or a painkiller to help combat our symptoms, without realizing what is actually going on.

So, one could just give up plant based foods in their diet, right? Unfortunately, lectins are found in every living thing. In fact, this protein is found in animal based products as well. Newer research shows that dairy products have the highest levels of lectin of all animal based foods. Fruits and vegetables are also not immune, as well as legumes, spices, oils, nuts, seeds, and sweeteners. This makes giving up lectin entirely an impossible task. To make matters worse, exact lectin content is largely unknown per specific food as this protein occurs naturally and his highly individualized. There are general ideas on high versus low lectin foods that can assist you in significantly decreasing your lectin intake.

The Science Behind Lectin

Lectins are a carbohydrate-binding protein that can attach to cell membranes. They become the 'communicator' for cells to organize and connect with their environment. There are several different types of lectins in various living organisms. In plants, lectins are primarily found in the roots and seeds, with the lowest level of lectin found in the leaves.

There are thousands of different types of lectins, many that have not been studied. Of those that have had the most research, 13 major classifications of lectin have emerged and their functions vary slightly, but two classes, agglutinins and prolamins, appear to cause the most damage to our bodies and are found in high lectin foods. Agglutinins and prolamins can have a major impact in how our gut and immune system functions often causing an inflammatory response.

When your intestinal wall is permeated or damaged by lectins, the protein leaks out into your bloodstream. At that time, the lectin can bind to glycoproteins that are found on the surface of most cells as well as to antibodies. The cells can be located anywhere in your body, including your joints, brain, liver, heart, and kidneys. Your body responds by attacking those cells which contains healthy material underneath. This triggering is known as an autoimmune response. Continual responses can lead to autoimmune diseases.

Where does gluten fit into all this?

You may now be wondering where gluten fits into all this, and you may be surprised to know that gluten is thought to be a type of lectin, specifically belonging to the prolamin class. This potentially means that while you're cutting gluten out of your diet, you're not actually resolving the issue. This is because other foods can contain lectin, not just those that also contain gluten. What this means is that even though you're cutting gluten out of your diet, you're perhaps not doing as much as you can to combat those nasty symptoms you suffer from. This may be why many people who have a gluten sensitivity who cut gluten from their diet still have symptoms, albeit to a lesser degree. Some of the highest lectin level foods contain gluten such as grains.

CHAPTER 2. WHY ARE LECTINS HARMFUL TO YOUR BODY?

There are many varieties of lectins and we have been researching them for over a hundred years. In fact, we have been using them as cell receptors in research studies for quite some time. Lectins are quite prolific. Polysaccharides (sugar molecules) cover the surface of most of the cells in your body and lectins bind to these molecules. Lectins are also resistant to the enzymes that break down our food in our stomach, allowing the lectin to pass through and stick to our intestinal walls. We know that lectins are directly linked to inflammation and subsequently autoimmune responses throughout your body.

Lectins, as we have already established, are a type of protein that helps the plant/animal/fish, defend itself against predators. If you or I ate a berry that made us feel ill afterward, it's likely that we would avoid eating it again. This is because the berry we consumed is likely to have contained a small amount of toxin, and we're likely to react to it slightly differently from one another, but it's likely to make us feel ill all the same.

Take the red kidney bean. You may have heard of Lectin Poisoning from this bean. Red kidney beans have a very high amount of lectin. If not cooked thoroughly, the high amount remains and the protein sticks to your red blood cells causing clotting issues that can make you very sick and can, in fact, cause death.

Why may we react differently?

You and I may react differently to foods that contain lectin as our bodies are slightly different. Let's say that you and I both eat that berry that I mentioned earlier, you may feel slightly nauseous, but I may have a bit of indigestion. Not many people are likely to react to the same thing in the same way. Take prescribed medication as an example: we've both been prescribed painkillers, but you get more benefit from them than I do. This is likely to be because our bodies contain different sensitivities, and simply react in a slightly different manner. It's how we are as humans, and it's one of life's mysteries.

Lectins and inflammation

Lectins are thought to cause inflammation, which can occur in the bloodstream, or inside your digestive tract. When this happens, we tend to experience a range of symptoms, depending on what we've eaten, how much we've eaten, and of course, how our body reacts to the food we've consumed.

19

The symptoms of the inflammation can include:

- Bloating

- Diarrhea

- Vomiting

- Stomachache

These symptoms can leave you feeling quite uncomfortable, again depending on how you react to them. Tackling these symptoms can often leave you feeling uncomfortable, tired, and achy. When you have a repeated amount of inflammation, over time, considerable damage can occur to your body and certain health problems such as autoimmune diseases could arise. In fact, some studies show that approximately 20% of Rheumatoid arthritis cases are caused by consuming lectins contained in the nightshade family (tomatoes, white potatoes, peppers).

Lectin and health conditions

There has been a fair amount of research into the causality of lectin and toxicity, but much more needs to occur before specific causality statements could be made. We do know that research has shown an association with the below conditions. Again, an association does not indicate causality and more research is needed. It is noted that the association could be that lectins could worsen the disease.

- ADHD
- Arthritis
- Asperger's
- Asthma
- Autism
- Cancer
- Congestive Heart Failure
- Crohn's disease
- Depression
- Diabetes type 1 & 2
- High blood pressure

- IBS

- Lupus

- Multiple sclerosis

- Obesity

- Rheumatoid arthritis

- Thyroiditis

- Parkinson's disease

- Polycystic ovary syndrome

- Premenstrual syndrome

- Ulcerative colitis

Lectins and the immune system

It's also thought that lectins may cause the immune system to work on over-drive. They do this by potentially encouraging the body to become sensitive to foods it wouldn't ordinarily be sensitive to. This could possibly mean that your lectin sensitivity could increase your

22

likelihood of developing lactose-intolerance, gluten-intolerance, or any other type of food intolerance.

Six Top Lectin Issues

Let's take a look at the overall top issues that research has shown lectin has a role in that could be curtailed with a reduced lectin diet.

1. Leaky gut- lectins bind to gut lining cells and when the lining becomes damaged, other proteins and bacteria enter your body also causing inflammation throughout your body. In fact, lectins can increase "bad" gut bacteria such as e. coli and decrease good bacteria such as iHSPs.

2. Autoimmune Responses- lectins increase inflammation which can lead to autoimmune responses and over time, chronic autoimmune diseases. Research on lectins have shown that they

stimulate class II HLA antigens including thyroid and pancreatic cells.

3. Obesity- lectin (specifically agglutin) can bind to cells that contain the hormone leptin. This hormone is responsible for telling your brain when you are full, fat metabolism, reproduction issues, immunity and growth. When lectin binds to the cells containing leptin, it disrupts the communication of leptin to your brain. Your brain does not get the appropriate message that you are full and overeating occurs. People who are obese have high levels of leptin.

4. Food sensitivity- lectins can cause your body to build up reactions to foods it finds toxic and can lead to food allergies. It is not surprising that the most common food allergies- peanuts, soy, dairy, eggs, wheat, tree nuts, shellfish, and fish are high in lectins.

5. Insulin-Agglutinin can cause insulin resistance and enlarge your pancreas which can reduce insulin levels.

6. Depression- many people discount the gut brain connection, but research shows there is a definite connection. In fact, those that suffer from Irritable Bowel Syndrome (IBS) have a 50-90% chance of also having a psychiatric disorder, including depression and/or anxiety. One reason this may be is the vagus nerve. This cranial nerve directly connects your gut to your brain and is responsible for, among many things, your gut communicating inflammation to your brain, breathing, your flight or fright response, and when your body needs to relax.

Evelyn Carmichael

CHAPTER 3. LOW AND HIGH LECTIN FOODS

If you were lactose-intolerant, you could easily avoid lactose by cutting out dairy products from your diet. If you knew you were simply gluten intolerant, you could cut out gluten from your diet. If you were allergic to nuts, you could make sure you never eat anything that contains nuts. However, the process of avoiding lectins is quite difficult, as they appear in many different foods, but you can reduce your lectin intake if you know which foods contain high quantities of this protein.

Lectin is found throughout nature and in most living plants, including the food we eat. Lectin is also located in nuts, seeds and spices. All fruits and vegetables contain some lectins, though there are some that contain higher levels including tomatoes and peppers.

Foods that contain high levels of lectin include Grains, Beans, Legumes, Grain Fed Meat and Dairy, and Nightshades.

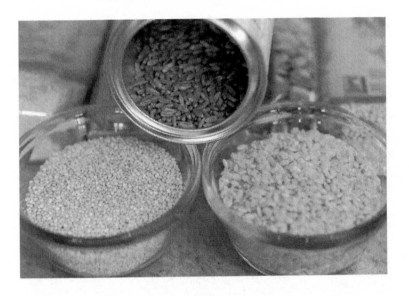

GRAINS

High Lectin
Wheat
Corn
Rye
Oats
Brown Rice
Barley
Millet
Quinoa
Spelt

Lower Lectin
Amaranth
Wild Rice
White Rice

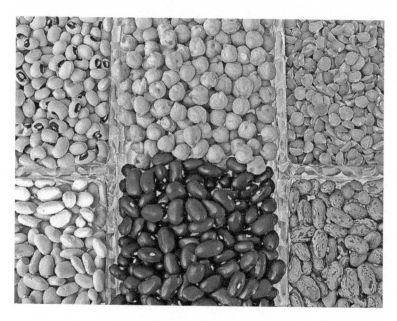

Legumes

Higher Lectin	**Lower Lectin**
Beans	None- but boiling,
Legumes	sprouting, fermenting,
Kidney Beans	or soaking legumes
Borlotti	helps reduce lectin
Soy	
Peanuts	
Peas	
Lentils	
Chickpeas	
Cacao Beans	

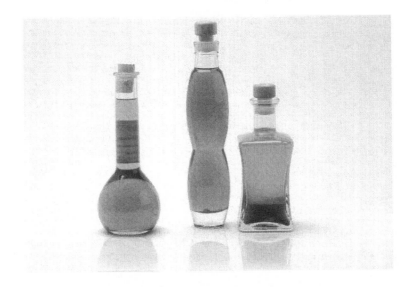

Oils

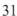

Higher Lectin	Lower Lectin
Grapeseed	Olive
Sunflower	Avocado
Peanut	Coconut
Corn	Sesame
Canola	Walnut
Cottonseed	Macadamia Nut
Safflower	Red Palm
	Rice Bran

31

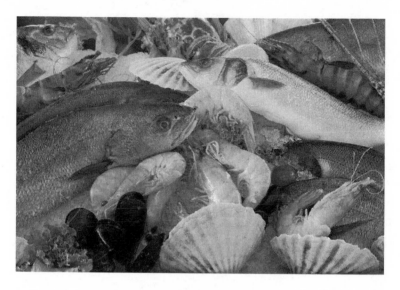

Seafood, Poultry, Meats

Higher Lectin	**Lower Lectin**
Grain Fed Meats and Poultry	Grass Fed Meats and Poultry & Fowl
	Eggs
	Turkey
	Ostrich
Grain Fed Dairy Products including milk, cheese, yogurt, cottage cheese, ice cream	Wild Caught Seafood
	Grass Fed Dairy Products

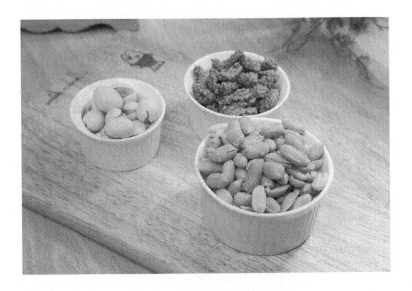

Nuts

Higher Lectin
Pine Nuts
Hazelnuts
Almonds
Cashews

Lower Lectin
Pecans
Walnuts
Pistachios
Macadamia
Chestnut

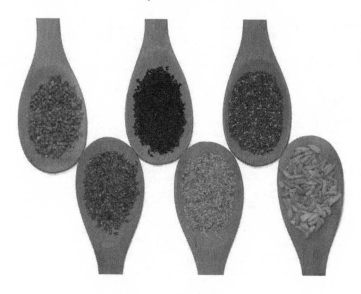

Seeds

<u>Higher Lectin</u>		**<u>Lower Lectin</u>**
Sesame		Pumpkin
Sunflower		Chia
		Hemp
		Flax

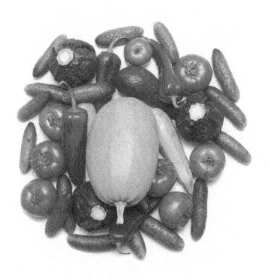

Nightshades

Higher Lectin	Lower Lectin
Tomatoes	Non-Nightshades like:
Corn/ Squash	Onions
Peppers	Mushrooms
Eggplant	Broccoli
White Potatoes	Cauliflower
Paprika/Tobacco/Garlic	Leafy Greens
Goji Berries	Bok Choy
Tomatillos	Asparagus
Okra/Pepinos	Avocado
Sorrel	Rhubarb
Capsicum	Carrots

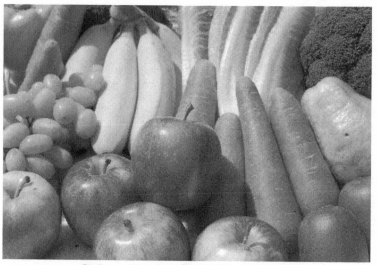

Other Fruits and Vegetables

<u>**Higher Lectin**</u>
Melons
Pumpkin
Corn

<u>**Lower Lectin**</u>
Bananas/Apples
Blueberries
Cherries
Kiwi/ Pineapple
Nectarines/Peaches
Oranges/Grapefruit
Strawberries/Raspberries
Celery/ Cucumbers
Leafy Greens- kale,
spinach, bib, radicchio,
chard, romaine, cabbage,
collard, greens

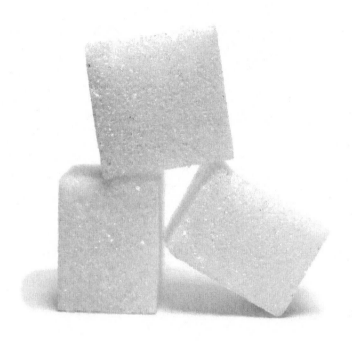

Sweeteners

Higher Lectin	**Lower Lectin**
Agave	Raw Honey
Sugar	Stevia
Sucralose	Xylitol
Artificial Sweeteners	Monk fruit
	Yacon

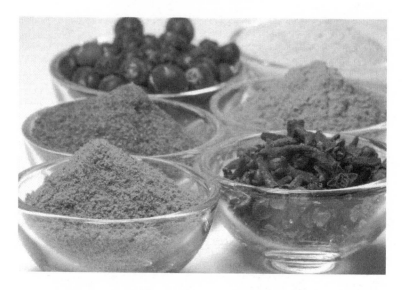

Spices

Higher Lectin	**Lower Lectin**
Peppermint	Black Pepper
Garlic	Vanilla
Nutmeg	Cinnamon
Marjoram	Most other spices
Caraway	have low lectin levels
Paprika/Chili Powder	

(Chart Notes: It is important to note that with Nightshades, there are not any low lectin alternatives specific to the nightshade family, however, you can prepare certain nightshades, namely beans/ legumes in a way that will reduce the natural lectin content. Tomatoes are another example where cooking can reduce the lectin content. This is explained in further detail in the next chapter.

Additionally, it is noted that since lectin is a naturally occurring protein, an exact amount is unable to be given. Lectin is calculated in a higher or lower range as it varies significantly and a numerical chart does not give an accurate picture. An example of this is the red kidney bean. Uncooked, the red kidney bean can vary from 20,000 to 70,000 hemagglutinating units.)

Evelyn Carmichael

CHAPTER 4. HOW TO REDUCE LECTIN COUNTS IN HIGH LECTIN FOODS

You will find that you can reduce the amount of lectin in your food by the way you prepare it. While some of these methods may be more time consuming than others, all these methods have been proven to reduce the lectin content and may be the difference between a food you can tolerate and one that causes inflammation or other nasty side effects due to its high lectin content.

Pressure Cooking

As you may know, pressure cooking decreases cooking time. By increasing the air pressure and the temperature, food is cooked in record time. Pressure cooking has been found to preserve the nutrition content of your food better than most any other cooking method. The added benefit is that this method destroys most lectins. In fact, if you soak legumes and then pressure cook them, you will destroy most of the lectins and will likely not have an adverse reaction to a previous high lectin content food!

Boiling

Similar to pressure cooking, boiling also reduces lectin content. Though with boiling alone, you cannot exceed the boiling point temperature of water as you can with pressure cooking. In order to reduce the amount of lectins in your foods you would need to make sure you boil for the full amount of cooking time.

Sprouting

One way for you to reduce your lectin intake, while also maintaining a diet rich in a variety of nutrients, is to sprout the beans, grains, and seeds that you eat. You may already consume these foods as part of your diet, but did you know that the longer you leave them to sprout the less lectin they contain?

The lectins can be found in the seed's coating, and as the seed starts to germinate the coat is metabolized, and it's this that helps to eliminate the lectins.

Why not think about growing sprouts at home, so you can enjoy them as and when you need them? It really is quite easy:

Line an unused tub or pot with some tissue paper, and sprinkle the seeds over, making sure they are evenly spread. Pour some water on, and leave in a sunny spot. Within a week you should start to see some growth. Allow the small sprouts to grow for at least a few weeks, ensuring that nasty lectin disappears.

If you do not have the time or desire to sprout your own seeds and grains, you may be able to find them in your store.

Milling and Rice

Rice is generally thought of as a gluten- free food, though in the grain family. For those with a lectin sensitivity, rice may not be the best choice, particularly brown rice for its high lectin value. White rice is a better option. It is milled from brown rice stripping the bran content. By milling the rice, it removes the lectin as well as phytic acid, which makes the rice more digestible and less harmful to the gut. While the nutrition may be less than that of brown rice, white rice is a safer bet for a starch that will not lead to inflammation.

Soak your beans and legumes

Another way to reduce your lectin intake is to soak your beans and legumes. Canned or uncooked beans and legumes can be soaked as well as rice. Not only will it reduce the amount of lectin, but you will also reduce naturally occurring arsenic. The cooking process of beans and legumes will also reduce the amount of lectin in each serving. Of course, they're likely to be cooked if they come in a can, but you can still reduce the amount of lectins further by rinsing and cooking again.

Here's where we can all make a difference to the foods that we eat:

Start buying raw beans and legumes. Not only are they cheaper, but you can cook most of the lectins out of them. Soak your beans and legume for about 8 hours, as this will help to reduce the lectins. Make sure you change the water frequently – I typically change the water every 2 hours, if I can, just to wash all the lectins away.

Once 8 hours is up, drain the water away, and rinse well. Now you're ready to cook your beans and legumes. One trick that I've learned along the way is to add a small amount of baking soda to the cooking water, as it helps to eliminate even more lectin. This includes red kidney beans. They have five times the amount of lectin in its uncooked form than cooked!

Cook your beans or legumes as required, but please make sure they are completely cooked before you end the cooking process. Once they're done, drain the water away, and rinse well. Your beans or legumes should now be ready to enjoy.

Fermenting

Fermenting is another way to reduce lectins. For example, fermented soy (i.e. miso) has much lower levels of lectin than its regular counterpart. Fermenting does not completely get rid of lectin levels, but it does help to reduce it.

How to ferment grains:

1. Take the amount of grains you would like to ferment and add enough water that you can easily stir but not be soupy.
2. Add buttermilk, whey, or kefir (enough to mix easily but not be soupy). Cover.
3. Place the mixture in a dry, warm place out of direct sunlight.
4. Let mixture sit covered for a minimum of 8 hours and a maximum of 24 hours.
5. After the time is up, uncover and drain excess liquid. Grains are ready to use.

Cooking

Similar to pressure cooking and boiling, simply cooking some of the high lectin foods will reduce the amount of lectins. A good example of this is tomatoes. A cooked tomato contains very low amounts of lectin. Peanuts, carrots, and grains are more resistant to heat and the lectins are unlikely to break down.

CHAPTER 5. REDUCING LECTIN FROM YOUR DIET

If you've now decided that you would like to reduce your intake of lectins, here are a few tips to get you started.

Run a trial period

Why not think about running a trial period whereby you reduce your lectin intake for the minimum of one week? Make a note of the foods you need to cut down on, make the necessary changes to your diet, and see how it goes. Of course, there may be a few hiccups along the way if you eat a food that does contain high amounts of lectin, but don't worry too much about it, just get back to the diet the next time you eat something.

Another method is to take one high lectin food per week and eliminate it from your diet and measure closely how you feel before removing another high lectin food. Remember, you could have a specific lectin sensitivity or a more broad ranging lectin intolerance and it may take some trial and error to get down to the culprit. There are antibody tests that can show certain types of lectin sensitivities, but they are not exhaustive by any means and most physicians and dieticians recommend closely monitoring your physical symptoms when removing high lectin foods.

Feeling better?

If you're feeling better for cutting down on your lectin, you may be onto something. Why not think about cutting down in the long term? Again, you can't ever have a lectin free diet, but you can strive to have a reduced lectin diet. If you are feeling better after removing some high lectin foods, you may want to continue down this path until your symptoms have dissipated. At that time, you may be able to occasionally have a high lectin food without having any associated symptoms. Remember, there are ways to eat high lectin foods by cooking them in a specific manner to remove most of the lectins.

Feeling the same?

If your trial period has made no difference to the way that you feel, try to think about what you could have done differently. While I do not encourage cutting out all lectin-containing foods, perhaps you still had a little too much in your diet. Give the trial another go, taking out another group of high lectin foods. An example would be say you decided to start your experiment by removing grains from your diet, but you still were experiencing the same symptoms that concern you 1-4 weeks later. Now, take another high lectin group out of your diet, say nightshades, and see how you feel a week after that.

Feeling worse?

Perhaps there are other underlying health issues. Please speak to your doctor as soon as you can, and ask for a blood test. An antibody test may be able to indicate if you have a specific intolerance to a small amount of lectin classifications that are able to be tested, though this may not be reliable due to the vast amount of lectins present in nature.

Change your diet gradually

If you have found that you feel better after your trial period, you may wish to start your new eating regime as soon as you can. The fact is that if you decide to cut down on lectin gradually, your change in diet will be much more sustainable.

Quite often when people begin new diets/eating regimes, they plunge into it feet first. They often tend to go 'the whole hog', without a thought, while assuming their new way of eating will be sustainable. As with any diet (and in particular quite restrictive ones), gradual changes are best. It's going to take your body about 4-6 weeks to get completely used to the ideal of a new way of eating. If you take the plunge and change your diet right away, you're setting yourself up for failure. Such changes are unsustainable as they will leave you craving the foods that you're used to eating.

Take time to gradually change what you eat, and your body and mind will thank you. Small changes will be easier to cope with, and you won't find that those nasty cravings are knocking at your door any time soon.

Make a note of the foods you like

If you have changed what you eat, if you've added new foods to your plan, or you've changed a recipe here and there, make a note of it, especially if you really like what you've eaten. If you make a note of the foods and meals that you know you enjoy eating, chances are you'll eat them again.

Enjoying what you eat means not only do you get to enjoy almost every mouthful, but it also means that this new eating regime of yours is likely to be more successful. So, make a note of those tasty dishes and treats, and enjoy them now and again.

Make a note of how much better you feel

For those with a lectin sensitivity, reducing or eliminating lectin will improve digestion and lead to less inflammation in your gut. As many know, your gut is an integral part of your body which can cause inflammation and flare-ups to many organs from your thyroid to your brain as well as your extremities.

One key factor for me when I was changing my diet was how I felt. I started to feel better and better as time went on, and I decided to make a note of this. You may have already gathered that I like making notes, but this was perhaps one of the most important ones I made. I noted how much more energy I had, how much better I felt within myself, and even how much better I slept. My energy level was higher throughout the day and I didn't have so much of that mid-afternoon slump that always made me yawn and want to crawl into bed.

Within the first two weeks of reducing lectin, I also noticed that my pants were looser, even though it wasn't part of the plan. At first I thought that I was just a little less bloated, but I somehow managed to lose a few pounds along the way, which was a nice bonus.

Making a note of how much better you feel can help you to stay on track, and keep your new eating regime going. Of course, there will be days when you make mistakes and eat something you perhaps should avoid, but give yourself a break, accept that it happens, and get back to it the next time you eat something.

CHAPTER 6. MAKING THE SWITCH TO LOW-LECTIN FOODS

When you start to make changes to the foods that you eat, you'll also need to start shopping differently. For example, those who have recently discovered they are lactose-intolerance will now need to look for foods that contain little or no lactose. This is the kind of thing you will have to do, you'll just have to look for the foods that contain little lectin.

Make a list of the high lectin foods you have decided to reduce or eliminate from your diet

These are the foods that you need to stay away from. Jot the list down on a bit of paper, or on your cell phone, and take it with you when you shop. Refer to the list when you're going around the store, and make sure you so that you don't accidentally buy something you need to avoid. Don't worry, after a while you'll start to learn which foods your body wants you to stay away from.

Think of the foods that you need to shop for

So, you've now decided that you would like to reduce your lectin intake, which means you may need to start shopping for foods that you've never eaten before, or not eaten very much of. Now is the time for you to write that grocery list, you may have gotten away with not having a list in the past, but now it's time for you to have one. This is because you're about to embark on a new eating regime that could include some nice new foods. It's unlikely that all of these foods will be at the forefront of your mind as you make your way around the store, so pre-planning some delicious new recipes and writing a list will help you stay on track.

Read the labels of all the products you buy

If you tend to buy any pre-packaged foods, bakery items, or prepared meals, you will want to read the ingredient labels before you buy. It's this list that will help you to determine whether you should or shouldn't buy the product in question. If you're not sure if you should buy it, refer to the list of the foods you are trying to cut down on and make sure it is not on the list. One of the good things about most items in the store these days is that the ingredient list is now clearly marked and in order of amount in the product you are buying.

Remember, you don't have to completely cut out lectin, this would be almost impossible, you just need to think about reducing your lectin intake.

Visit health food stores

If you don't usually frequent your local health food stores, I encourage you to do so. Take a look, and see what they have in stock. Remember, you are never under any obligation to buy anything, but it could be useful to see the range of products they have, just in case you can't get the things you need in your local supermarket.

Be warned, some products may be more expensive in health food stores, so you may want to see if you can get them elsewhere. It always pays to shop around, as there are usually different bargains to be had in different stores. Plus, shopping around could potentially mean that your diet is full of a wide variety of foods, and that's never a bad thing! Local supermarkets are changing to more healthy alternatives as well and may well have a very large selection of foods that will fit in to your reduced lectin diet.

Start to cook from scratch

I am a great advocate for home cooked meals. You know exactly what has gone into them, and you can control what you *don't* put in. Plus, home cooked meals usually taste better, and they usually turn out to be cheaper too – especially if you work out how much the meal costs per portion.

Make the changes as soon as you can

There's not been as much research in the lectin world as there has been in the gluten world, but it is thought that lectin could contribute to a number of health conditions. More research is continuing in the gluten free diet versus reduced lectin realm, but until then, you can do what you can to make yourself feel better.

Lectins are everywhere, so if you believe you have a lectin sensitivity, it is important to think about this as a Lectin Reduction or Avoidance Diet not a Lectin Elimination Diet. You can try to avoid high lectin foods or prepare them in a manner to reduce the amount of lectins in them. It is unrealistic to think you can completely eliminate lectins from your diet, but you can make significant changes to the amount you are exposed to.

Many people who have a lectin sensitivity are able to reduce the amount to the point they are not having flare ups or symptoms they were having before. In fact, many anecdotal studies have reported that those that limit their lectin intake can occasionally have high lectin foods without causing the symptoms they have had before.

Making these much-needed changes may help you to feel so much better. You may be less bloated, less uncomfortable, and you may even sleep better at night. Just think, a few changes to the foods that you eat could make a few significant changes to your health, leaving you feeling and looking so much better.

If you want to improve your digestive system, reduce inflammation, and ultimately improve your health, reducing your lectin intake may be the key to feeling better every single day.

Read on for an excerpt of Evelyn Carmichael's book *The Essential Handbook to Turmeric and Ginger*, **now on Amazon.**

Evelyn Carmichael

THE ESSENTIAL HANDBOOK TO TURMERIC AND GINGER

THE ANTI-INFLAMMATORY DUO THAT WILL CHANGE YOUR LIFE

By
EVELYN CARMICHAEL

Evelyn Carmichael

INTRODUCTION

Many of us are more than happy to rely on prescribed medication to help us cure a wide variety of ills. But did you know that people all over the world have been using spices to help relieve and even cure a variety of conditions?

Turmeric and ginger are two of the most powerful and commonly used spices that are known to fight inflammation, infections, and so much more.

Even though we in the western world are used to taking prescribed medications, some of us are just starting to discover the real benefits of these ancient yet highly nutritious spices.

Let this book show you the benefits of turmeric and ginger. Discover how you too can use the natural power of these spices to help you feel better and prevent a variety of ailments.

Let this book also show you how to use these ancient spices, and learn how to cook a few delicious meals and treats, that can help you benefit from the way they work.

Evelyn Carmichael

CHAPTER 1. THE HEALTH BENEFITS OF TURMERIC

Turmeric is thought to be one of the healthiest spices you'll come across. This spice, like ginger, contains a wide range of nutrients and compounds, and has incredible anti-inflammatory properties.

Turmeric's origin is from a plant found in southern Asia and India is still the world's largest source of the flavorful spice. In fact, it is the main spice used to make curry. But the root of the turmeric plant is the source of which medicine, food colorings, and even cosmetics can be originated from. With an active compound known as curcumin, this spice really has a lot going for it

Let's take a close look at just some of the health benefits of this wonderful spice:

Anti-inflammatory properties and absorption

Turmeric naturally contains over two dozen anti-inflammatory properties that can help to reduce swelling. Curcumin may well be the most powerful of the bunch, but is hard to get the amount you need and for your body to absorb it in the amounts found in curry recipes. To get the full benefits of the curcumin in Turmeric, it is recommended to use turmeric extract. Furthermore, recent studies have shown that to better absorb the turmeric extract, taking it with black pepper is extremely beneficial. While swallowing a couple of peppercorns may seem strange to you, be aware that some studies show absorption rates increasing to 2000%. Lately, you can find Turmeric (or labeled as curcumin) with black pepper together as an extract in the health food store.

Managing arthritis

Those who suffer from arthritis are frequently in pain, and turmeric can help. Thanks to the active properties found in curcumin, it can be used to help combat the associated pain and discomfort sufferers often feel. Incredibly, those who had taken curcumin as part of a trial were found to have a little less pain, and other symptoms.

Anticoagulant properties

Turmeric is thought to work as an anticoagulant by preventing platelets from sticking together, turmeric prevents blood clots from forming and remaining. This in turn, will help prevent heart attacks and strokes. Please speak to your doctor before you decide to use turmeric as an anticoagulant.

Antidepressant

Incredibly, it's thought that this lovely-tasting spice can work as an antidepressant. When used as part of a study in a laboratory, and on animals who were considered to be depressed, it was found that turmeric helped to relieve some of their symptoms. Furthermore, when this spice was used in human patients, it was thought that it has the same effect as Prozac when it comes to managing depression.

Lowering blood sugar levels

Adding a little bit of turmeric to your diet is thought to help reduce blood sugar levels in those with type 2 diabetes. It's also considered to be effective at helping to reverse some of the side effects that are associated with hyperglycemia, and insulin resistance. Those with type 2 diabetes should consider adding a little turmeric to their diet each day.

Alleviating pain

Turmeric extract is thought to have more anti-inflammatory agents that help relieve pain then many over the counter pain killers. In fact, many people use turmeric extract instead of an aspirin or other painkiller. While you should always take any pain medication that has been prescribed by your doctor, knowing that turmeric can help means you may be in a little less pain very soon.

Evelyn Carmichael

Lowering cholesterol levels

We all know that the foods we consume can have a direct impact on our cholesterol levels. The good news is that turmeric can help to lower those levels. A study that took place, whereby individuals with high cholesterol were given turmeric showed that when they consumed turmeric daily, their cholesterol levels reduced slightly. In fact, several studies have shown that not only does turmeric extract reduce "bad" cholesterol, it also reduces the plaque buildup in your arteries which is a significant cause of many heart issues and strokes.

Please note that if your doctor has prescribed you cholesterol-reducing medication, you should still take it.

Gastrointestinal issues

Anyone who suffers from gastrointestinal issues such as Crohn's disease, irritable bowel syndrome, or ulcerative colitis should consider consuming turmeric every day. The curcumin that's found in turmeric is thought to relieve the pain and discomfort experienced in these conditions, as well as acting as an anti-inflammatory. In some individuals who regularly consumed turmeric, it was found that they no longer needed to take the corticosteroids that were prescribed.

Please make sure you continue to take any mediation that your doctor prescribes you, even if you're feeling better.

Liver damage

Studies have shown that increasing your intake of curcumin each day could help to delay cirrhosis. This is all thanks to the anti-inflammatory and antioxidant effect that curcumin has. Those who currently suffer from liver damage should continue taking any mediation that has been prescribed to them by their doctor.

Alzheimer's Disease

Turmeric has also been shown to have positive uses in managing Alzheimer's Disease. Curcumin can speed up the clearance of amyloid protein plaques, reducing and the progression and symptoms of Alzheimer's.

To find out more of the amazing benefits and uses for Turmeric and Ginger, please visit https://www.amazon.com/dp/B01N2B8KBN.

Evelyn Carmichael

ABOUT THE AUTHOR

Evelyn Carmichael

Evelyn was in the world of corporate finance before switching her life path after a successful battle with breast cancer. She is a personal life coach, fitness guru, and healthy lifestyle advocate.

Find out more on Facebook or at https://www.amazon.com/Evelyn-Carmichael/e/B01MQYHZLC

Evelyn Carmichael

OTHER BOOKS BY EVELYN CARMICHAEL

Evelyn is the author of the Essential Handbook Series.

Her titles include the following:

Healthy Diet Plans for Health Issues:

The Essential Handbook to a Healthy Gut

The Essential Handbook to the High Fiber Diet

The Essential Handbook to the Alzheimer's Diet

The Essential Handbook to Reversing Prediabetes and Diabetes: Meal Plans and Recipes to Reduce Your Blood Sugar Levels and Eliminate Diabetes and Prediabetes

The Essential Handbook to Hashimoto's

The Essential Handbook for Choosing the Right Diet: A Guide to the Most Popular Diets and if They are Right for You

Evelyn Carmichael

Anti-Inflammation and Super Foods:

The Essential Handbook to Superfood Smoothies

The Essential Handbook to Avocados The Superfood that Reduce Inflammation and lowers blood sugar, blood pressure, and your cholesterol

The Essential Handbook to Turmeric and Ginger: The Anti-Inflammatory Duo that will Change your Life

The Essential Handbook to Coconut Oil: Tips, Recipes, and How to use for weight loss and in your daily life

The Essential Handbook to Apple Cider Vinegar: Tips and Recipes for Weight Loss and Improving your Health, Beauty, & Home

Instant Pot Cookbooks:

The Essential Handbook to Diabetic Instant Pot Cooking

The Essential Handbook to Gluten Free Instant Pot Cooking

The Essential Handbook to Paleo Instant Pot Cooking

The Essential Handbook to Lectin

<u>Healthy Living:</u>

The Essential Handbook to Herbal Remedies

The Essential Handbook to Hygge

The Art of Keeping Goals

The Essential Handbook to Natural Living

The Essential Handbook to Essential Oils: Tips and Recipes for Weight Loss, Stress Relief, and Pain Management

Knee Supports: Uses, Exercises, and Benefits

Evelyn Carmichael

REFERENCES

1. http://www.ncbi.nlm.nih.gov/pubmed/25599185
2. http://www.whfoods.com/genpage.php?pfriendly=1&tname=foodspice&dbid=87
3. http://ajcn.nutrition.org/content/33/11/2338.long
4. http://www.ncbi.nlm.nih.gov/pubmed/8777015
5. http://www.ncbi.nlm.nih.gov/pmc/articles/PMC1382815/
6. https://link.springer.com/article/10.1007/BF00494350
7. http://www.ncbi.nlm.nih.gov/pubmed/10884708
8. http://www.ncbi.nlm.nih.gov/pmc/articles/PMC2271815/
9. https://www.ncbi.nlm.nih.gov/pmc/articles/PMC1115436/
10. http://www.ncbi.nlm.nih.gov/pubmed/7407532
11. http://poisonousplants.ansci.cornell.edu/toxicagents/lectins.html
12. http://www.ncbi.nlm.nih.gov/pmc/articles/PMC1933252/
13. http://www.ncbi.nlm.nih.gov/pubmed/16441922
14. https://www.ncbi.nlm.nih.gov/pmc/articles/PMC2271815/pdf/epidinfect00024-0031.pdf

Evelyn Carmichael

AUTHOR NOTE

If you enjoyed this book, found it useful or otherwise then I'd really appreciate it if you would post a short review on Amazon. I do read all the reviews personally so that I can continually write what people are wanting.

Thanks for your support!

Evelyn Carmichael

Made in the USA
San Bernardino, CA
28 September 2017